SENSS Enterprises

Ten steps to five

Staffordshire County Council & The Questions Publishing Company, 2000

First published 1997
This edition 2000

This edition published by
The Questions Publishing Company Ltd
27 Frederick Street, Birmingham B1 3HH
Tel: 0121 212 0919   Fax:0121 212 0959
Website: www.education-quest.com

Designed by Al Stewart
Illustrations and cover design by Steven Molloy

Original design by
SENSS Enterprises
Special Educational Needs Support Service
Flash Ley Resource Centre
Hawksmoor Road
STAFFORD
ST17 9DR
Tel: 01785-356853
Fax: 01785-356854

Contents

Acknowledgements

Compiled by

Gill Mansell
Nola Wilde
SENSS

Pat Djemli and the Staff Team of
Tamworth Day Nursery

Norma Francis and the Staff Team of
Stafford Day Nursery

.

Key principles behind the assessment of *under fives*

Often with pre-school children there may be a number of professionals involved, each reporting on the same aspect of the child (e.g. the child with limited language may be working with a psychologist, nursery teacher, speech therapist, school medical officer, social worker and parents) and assessment may be fragmented with each professional holding one piece of the overall picture.

"The first principle of all assessment, and especially pre-school, must be to provide a whole picture, not a series of disjointed images."

(*Support for Learning* Vol. 5, No 2, 1990)

Promoting children's learning is a principal aim of schools.

"Assessment lies at the heart of this process. It can provide a framework in which educational objectives may be set, and pupil's progress charted and expressed. It can yield a basis for planning the next educational steps in response to children's needs."

(National Curriculum TGAT, para. 3, 1988)

Teachers have long appreciated the value of early identification of potential learning difficulties. The Bullock Report in 1975 recommended a systematic procedure for the "prevention and treatment of learning difficulties" and the 1981 Education Act established the same framework for under fives as it did for older children.

With the advent of National Curriculum, the concepts of national testing at 7, 11, 14 and baseline assessment . . .

". . . it is (thought to be) highly advisable that the process of continuous

assessment should begin at an earlier stage than Key Stage 1. Intervention to prevent learning failure should be initiated rapidly and monitored continuously through the school years. Schools will now be more accountable for learning failure and it will become increasingly important that they can demonstrate the steps of early identification and remediation if they are to maximise learning opportunities for all children."

(EYES)

Areas of development

This developmental record has not been envisaged as the traditional pass/fail type, but rather to be used as a tool to evaluate progress, plan curriculum and to obtain an overall picture of the child.

After much discussion it was decided to divide the record into five main areas in which some form of assessment and remediation would be appropriate. These categories help give a picture of the strengths and weaknesses of the whole child.

1 **Posture and large movements**
"The development of good motor skills, both gross and fine, is fundamental to overall development and essential for good learning ability."
(Early Learning Assessment and Development)

2 **Vision and fine movements**
"Associated with the development of motor skills is the growth of body awareness and the child's perception of his position in space."

"A child's ability to co-ordinate his eye-hand movements and perceive himself, both in space and in relation to others, is dependent upon the development of an adequate body image."

"Visual perception is involved in almost every action."

"Accurate visual perceptual skills are needed for reading, writing, spelling and mathematics."

(Early Learning Assessment and Development)

3 Hearing and speech

"Auditory competence (must be) determined as well as use of language codes."

(From Birth to Five Years – Mary Sheridan)

"Effective communication is of prime importance in any learning situation as without the ability to use language all but the most basic levels of learning are impossible."

"Communication can be both verbal and non-verbal."

"In everyday life auditory discrimination becomes essential since the meaning of what is heard by a child depends upon his ability to distinguish between fine differences in sound, e.g. make or take."

(Early Learning Assessment and Development)

4 Social and emotional behaviour

"In the assessment of social behaviour, it is necessary to seek evidence not only regarding capability in self-care (dressing, feeding, toilet, etc.) but also regarding the child's ability to establish good personal relationships, his general understanding of everyday situations and his willingness to conform to reasonable social demands."

"Basic psychological needs relate both to intellectual and emotional development . . . They include:

● *affection and continuity of individual care;*

- *security rooted in a knowledge of belonging, in stable personal relationships and in familiar environmental conditions;*

- *a sense of personal identity, dignity as a human being, and self-respect derived from knowledge of being valued as an individual;*

- *opportunity to learn from experience;*

- *opportunity to achieve success in some field of endeavour, however small;*

- *opportunity to take responsibility, however slight, and to be of service to others."*

(From Birth to Five Years – Mary Sheridan)

5   Play

*"It is the nature of the developing **body** to be continually active, of the developing **mind** to be intensely curious and of the developing **personality** to seek good relationships with other people."*

(From Birth to Five Years – Mary Sheridan)

Aims of this record of achievement

- To highlight a child's strengths as well as weaknesses, enabling teachers to plan the curriculum accordingly.

- To use common play materials and everyday nursery procedures and strategies. No expensive equipment is necessary.

- To be quick and easy to use.

- To be purposeful, clear and unambiguous.

- To be an informal approach to assessment, enabling children to be observed in natural situations.

- To provide an accurate record of achievement for parents and staff.

- To co-ordinate information and be freely available to all professionals involved.

Some observations described in the left hand column of the record sheets may require:

a)   *an intervention to develop a particular skill*

b)   *an intervention to modify inappropriate behaviour*

c)   *a tick and/or a dated comment*

d)   *no comment needed*

Presentation and general usage

"The manner of the child's response is usually more illuminating than the mere fact of his ability or inability to comply with the instruction."

Mary Sheridan

One of the main concerns of Early Years personnel in the use of checklists is that they either do not give enough space for comments or they require too much irrelevant information. Often, allowance needs to be made for distractibility due to excitement, or timidity or anxiety, for grief following separation from family and home, also for the nature of the child's social environment and the opportunities to learn from experience.

The chart used allows three large areas for date/comment, and additional boxes for further comment which can be copied on to the back of sheets when/if required.

For the sake of brevity, the child is referred to as he throughout the record.

Only one or two sheets per child for each main area is required.

It is envisaged that this will be a 'rolling record' whereby staff will update one area each week, working though all five categories, i.e. total update every 5/6 weeks.

Each child will then have an ongoing Record of Achievement throughout his time in the nursery.

Step 1
The first 3 months

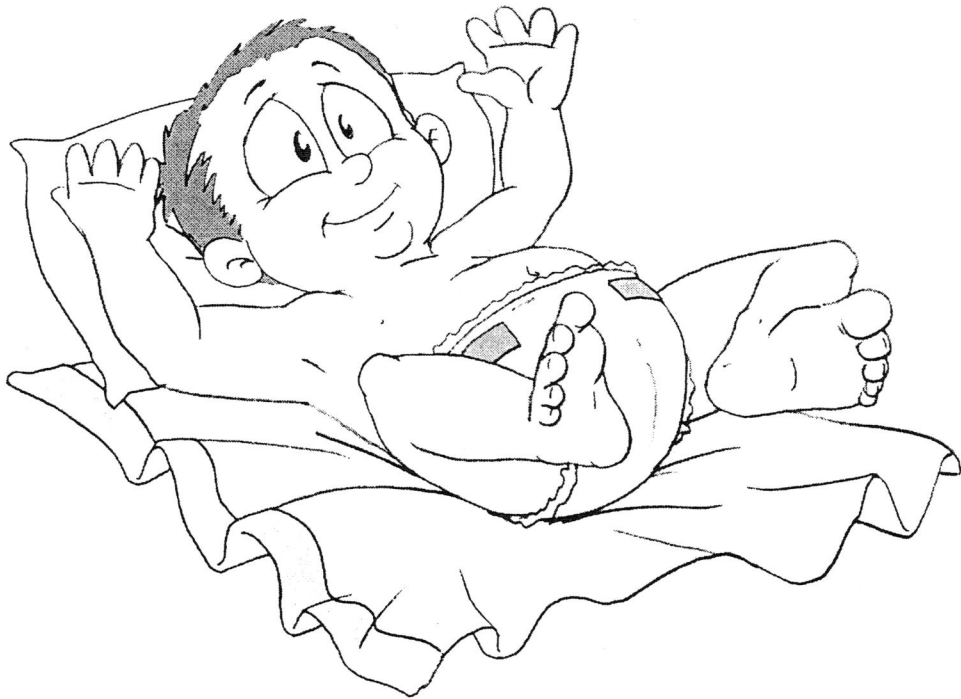

Posture and Large Movements (Step 1)

Observation	Date first noted	Action Taken	Date Checked
Arms more active than legs.			
When held in sitting position head falls forward.			
Makes reflex stepping movements when held in a standing position.			
Kicks vigorously.			
If placed downwards on face, may lift head and upper chest using arms to support.			
When held in sitting position, back is straight - little or no head lag.			
Holds rattle for a few moments.			

Vision and Fine Movements (Step 1)

Observation	Date first noted	Action Taken	Date Checked
Hands tightly clenched and will only open when touched.			
Grasps finger.			
Turns head towards light.			
Follows light briefly with eyes.			
Shuts eyes tightly when bright light is shone directly into them.			
Eyes follow dangling toy 6 - 10 inches from face.			
Looks at mother's face whilst feeding from about three weeks.			
Begins to clasp and unclasp hands together in finger play.			
Visually very alert - near and far.			
Follows adult movements with head and eyes.			

Vision and Fine Movements (Step 1) - continued

Observation	Date first noted	Action Taken	Date Checked
Very interested in human faces.			
Watches movement of own hands.			

Hearing and Speech (Step 1)

Observation	Date first noted	Action Taken	Date Checked
Head turns to speaker.			
Attends to meaningful sounds.			
Coos, when content.			
When spoken to shows excitement and vocalises.			

Social and Emotional Behaviour (Step 1)

Observation	Date first noted	Action Taken	Date Checked
Sleeps most of the time when not being fed or handled.			
Sucks well.			
Becoming more alert, progressing to a social smile and responsive vocalisation.			
When picked up and spoken to stops crying.			
Cries lustily when hungry or uncomfortable.			
Coos responsively to mother's talk.			
Recognises feeding bottle.			
Engages in finger play.			
Fixes eyes unblinkingly on mother's face when feeding.			
Enjoys caring routines.			

Social and Emotional Behaviour (Step 1) - continued

Observation	Date first noted	Action Taken	Date Checked
Responds with obvious pleasure to friendly handling.			
Responds well to playful tickling.			

Play (Step 1)

Observation	Date first noted	Action Taken	Date Checked
Learns to attract mother's attention by vigorous movements, smiles and coos when handled or talked to.			
Hand and eye co-ordination - interlacing finger play.			
Able to open and shut hands and scratch surface upon which he lies appreciating resulting sight and sound.			
Will clasp a toy firmly, bringing it towards his face although he may bang himself in the process.			
May be able to hold rattle between two hands clasping and unclasping alternately.			
May be able to drop rattle or toy by opening hands, but cannot yet place it down neatly and deliberately.			
Likely to discover feet - foot/eye co-ordination develops.			

Step 2
3 – 6 months

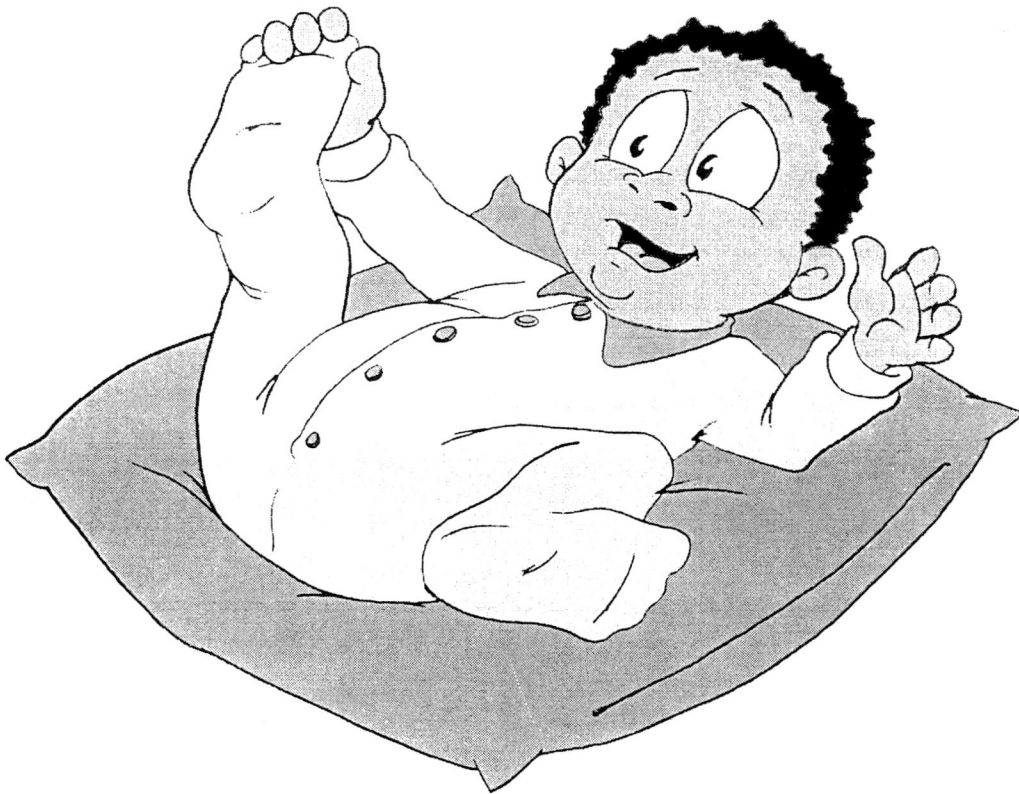

Posture and Large Movements (Step 2)

Observation	Date first noted	Action Taken	Date Checked
Lifts legs and grasps foot.			
Sits with support.			
Holds arms up to be lifted.			
Can roll over front to back.			
When held in sitting position, head held firmly erect and back straight.			
When held under arms in standing position bears weight on feet and bounces up and down.			

Vision and Fine Movements (Step 2)

Observation	Date first noted	Action Taken	Date Checked
Uses whole hand to grasp objects.			
Moves head and eyes eagerly in every direction to see objects and people.			
Eyes move in unison.			
Smooth following eye movements in all directions.			

Hearing and Speech (Step 2)

Observation	Date first noted	Action Taken	Date Checked
Chuckles and squeals aloud at play.			
Makes tuneful noises to self and others.			
Cries to attract attention.			
Screams with annoyance.			

Social and Emotional Behaviour (Step 2)

Observation	Date first noted	Action Taken	Date Checked
Turns immediately to mother's voice across the room.			
Still friendly with strangers but occasionally shows shyness.			
Laughs and chuckles and squeals aloud in play.			
Screams with annoyance.			
Shows evidence of selective responses to different emotional notes in mother's voice.			

Play (Step 2)

Observation	Date first noted	Action Taken	Date Checked
Able to reach for and grasp rattle and look at it with a prolonged gaze.			
Able to shake rattle.			
Able to take rattle to mouth and withdraw it.			
Uses two hands and, a little later, two feet together.			
Able to hold two objects, one in each hand, and bring them together to meet.			
Able to pass toy from one hand to the other with voluntary hand release.			

Step 3
6 – 12 months

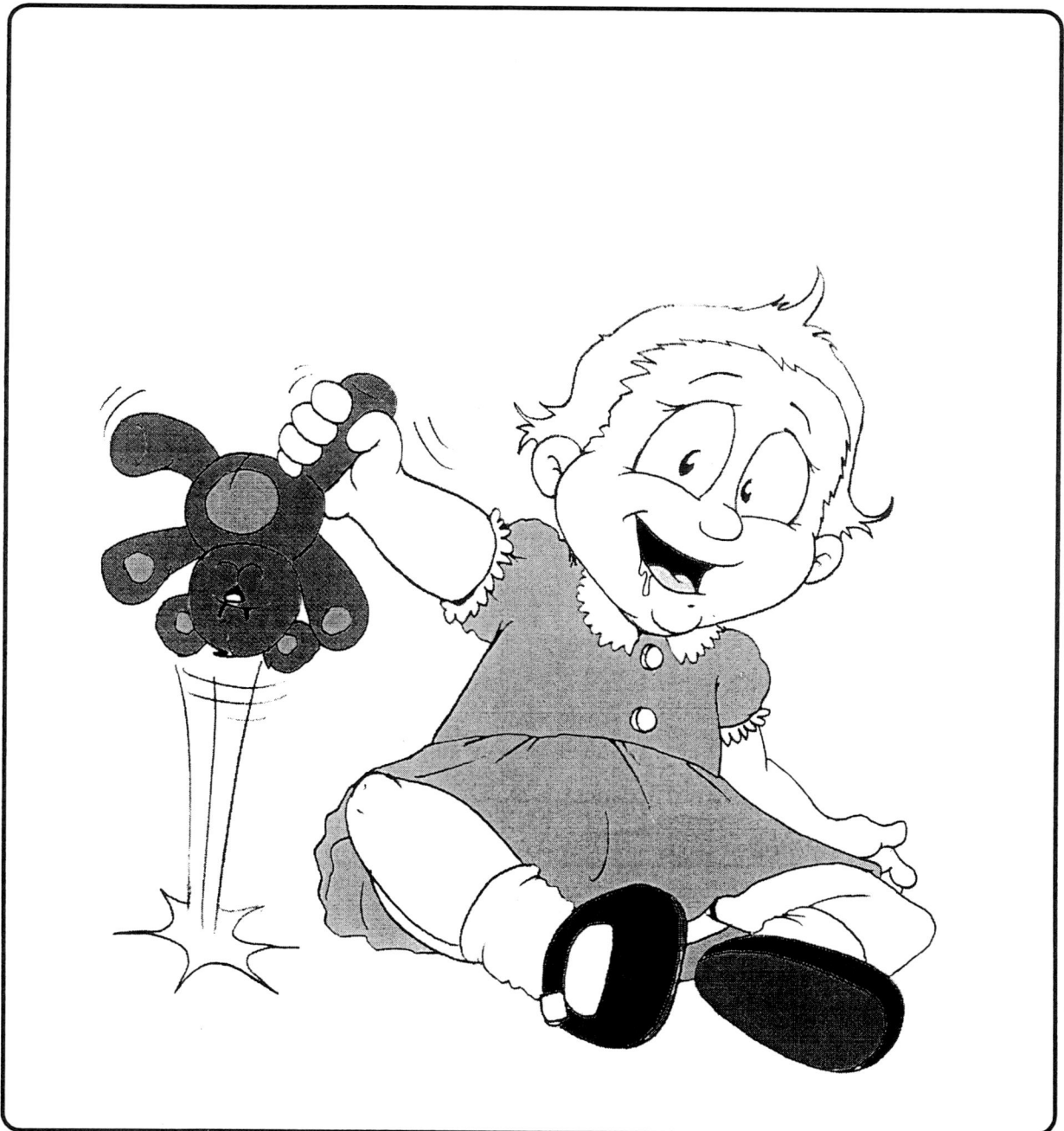

Posture and Large Movements (Step 3)

Observation	Date first noted	Action Taken	Date Checked
Can sit alone for 10-15 minutes.			
Attempts to crawl.			
Sometimes pulls self to standing position, with support.			
If held in standing position, steps purposefully on alternate feet.			

Vision and Fine Movements (Step 3)

Observation	Date first noted	Action Taken	Date Checked
Pokes at small objects with index finger.			
Grasps sweets, string etc. between fingers and thumb in inferior pincer grasp.			
Sometimes pulls self to standing position, with support.			
Passes objects from hand to hand.			
Very observant.			
Watches activities of adults, children and animals within 2-3 metres with eager interest.			

Hearing and Speech (Step 3)

Observation	Date first noted	Action Taken	Date Checked
Babbles long repetitive strings of syllables (da-da, ba-ba).			
Imitates adult's playful sounds including occasional word forms.			
Understands and knows few words, e.g. 'No' and 'Bye bye'.			
Joins up a variety of unrecognisable but different sounds into sentences.			

Social and Emotional Behaviour (Step 3)

Observation	Date first noted	Action Taken	Date Checked
Plays 'peek-a-boo' and clasps hands.			
Understands 'No' and 'Good-bye'.			
Clearly distinguishes strangers from familiar faces.			
Throws back body and stiffens with annoyance.			
Clings to known adults and hides face.			

Play (Step 3)

Observation	Date first noted	Action Taken	Date Checked
Able to reach out for toys at arm's length without falling over when sitting.			
Creeps towards eye-catching objects.			
Throws toys about and watches and listens with satisfaction to resulting movement and noise.			
Shows pleasure banging small objects on hard surfaces.			
Looks at a new toy for a few minutes before reaching for it.			
Recognising permanence of objects and will search for a toy if hidden.			
Is able to concentrate on one toy at a time.			

Step 4
12 – 18 months

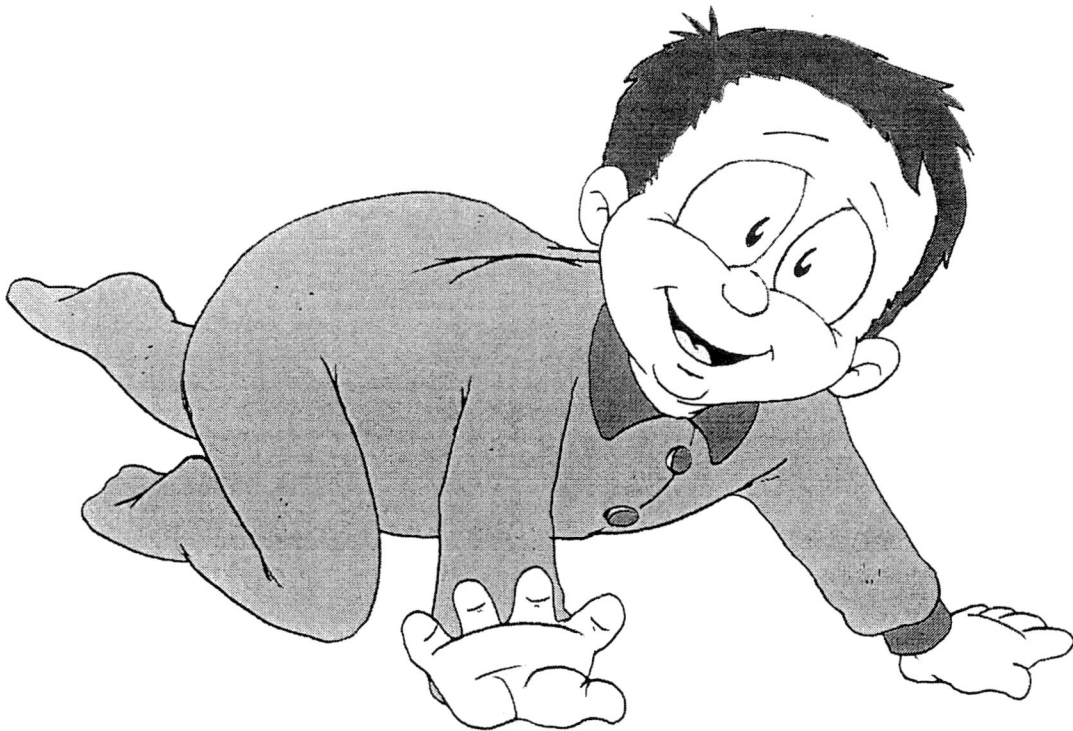

Posture and Large Movements (Step 4)

Observation	Date first noted	Action Taken	Date Checked
Rises to sitting position from lying down.			
Crawls on hands and knees or shuffles on bottom.			
Crawls upstairs.			
Sometimes walks round furniture.			
Walks unevenly - feet wide apart and arms held out to balance.			
Walks alone.			
Climbs on furniture and needs help to get down.			

Vision and Fine Movements (Step 4)

Observation	Date first noted	Action Taken	Date Checked
Picks up small objects such as sweets and string with precise grasp of thumb and index finger.			
Points with index finger at objects which interest.			
Picks up objects using either hand.			

Hearing and Speech (Step 4)

Observation	Date first noted	Action Taken	Date Checked
Alert to very quiet meaningful sounds but soon becomes quite bored when sound repeated without an interesting result.			
Turns to voice appropriately.			
Speaks 2-6 words and understands many more.			
Points to familiar persons, animals, toys that he wants.			
Understands and obeys simple commands (e.g. 'Fetch your shoes').			
Knows and turns to own name, and may recognise a few other names.			
Uses sound deliberately to communicate.			
Shouts to attract attention, listens and then shouts again.			

Social and Emotional Behaviour (Step 4)

Observation	Date first noted	Action Taken	Date Checked
Drinks from a cup with a little assistance, sitting in one place.			
Can chew.			
Holds spoon but cannot yet use it alone.			
Helps with dressing by holding out arm for sleeve and foot for shoe.			
Likes to be within sight and hearing of familiar adult.			
Plays 'pat-a-cake' and waves 'bye-bye' on request.			
Demonstrates affection to familiar people.			
Needs constant supervision to protect from danger in his environment.			

Play (Step 4)

Observation	Date first noted	Action Taken	Date Checked
Begins to enjoy 'give and take' play.			
Begins to imitate.			
Demonstrates 'definition by use' in relation to common objects, e.g. brings a cup to his lips or a brush to his hair.			
Able to manipulate blocks with a good pincer grip but seldom aligns more than three on the flat or in a tower whether in imitation or spontaneously.			
Enjoys activities which make a noise, e.g. tearing paper or playing with percussion instruments.			
Begins to sort, with adult help.			
Mouthing of toys becomes less.			
Enjoys combining two toys in an active way, e.g. banging two blocks together. He is also able to carry them.			

Play (Step 4) - continued

Observation	Date first noted	Action Taken	Date Checked
Explores the play possibilities of the home environment and constant supervision becomes necessary as he becomes more mobile.			

Step 5
18 months – 2 years

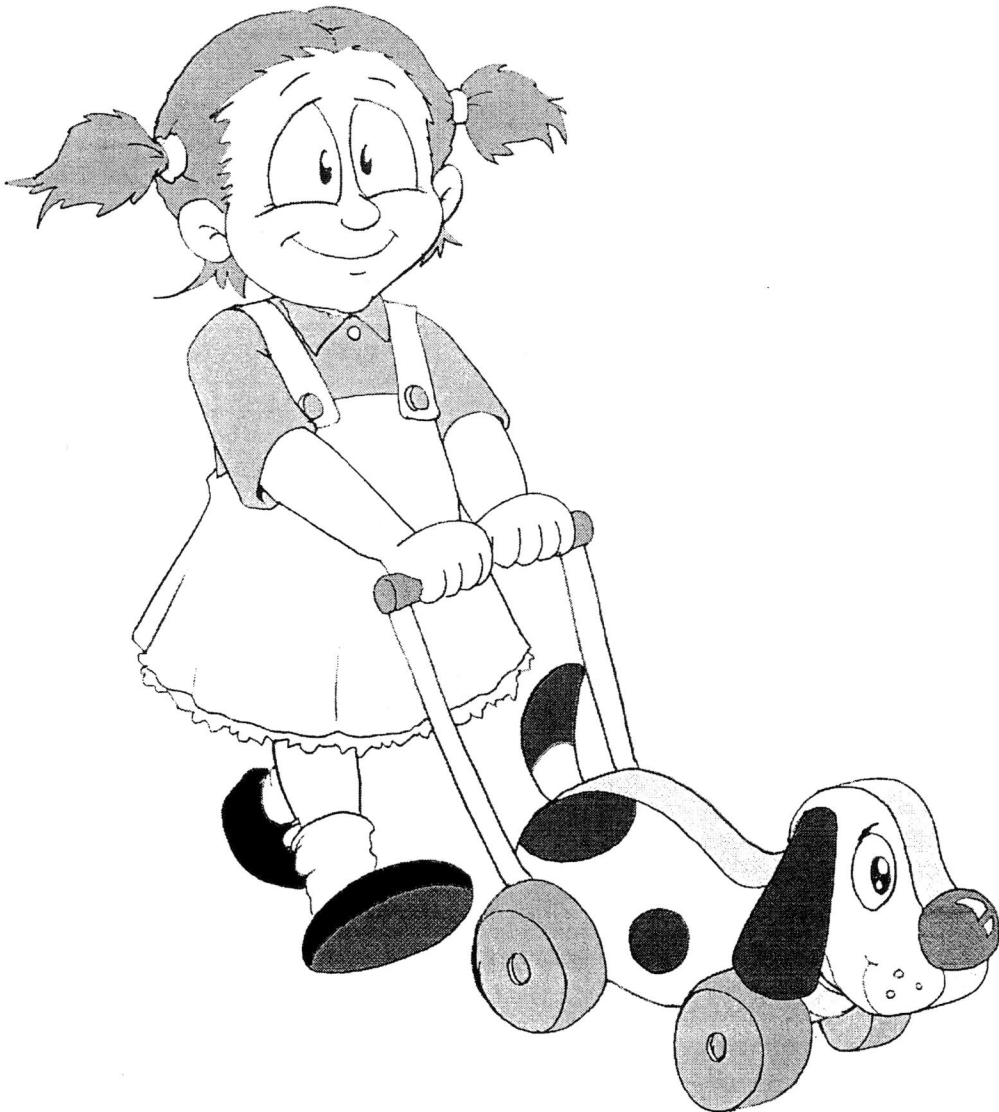

Posture and Large Movements (Step 5)

Observation	Date first noted	Action Taken	Date Checked
Walks well, carrying toy.			
Starts and stops safely.			
Runs carefully but cannot continue around obstacles.			
Pushes and pulls large wheeled toys, boxes etc. around floor.			
Backs into small chair or slides in sideways.			
Climbs forward on to adult chair.			
Walks up and down stairs with help.			
Squeals to pick up fallen toy.			
Kneels upright on flat surface.			

Vision and Fine Movements (Step 5)

Observation	Date first noted	Action Taken	Date Checked
Able to pick up small sweets, beads, etc. with neat pincer grasp.			
Holds pencil in mid-shaft.			
Able to scribble spontaneously.			
Able to build a tower of three cubes after demonstration.			
Enjoys simple picture books, often recognising and pointing to boldly coloured objects.			
When sharing a book, will turn several pages at a time.			

Hearing and Speech (Step 5)

Observation	Date first noted	Action Taken	Date Checked
Chatters loudly and continually to himself at play.			
Attends when speech addressed directly to him.			
Able to use 6 - 20+ recognisable words and understands many more.			
Indicates needs and wants by use of words and gestures.			
Enjoys nursery rhymes and attempts to join in.			
Imitates actions in action rhymes.			
Offers named familiar objects correctly when requested.			
Responds to simple one-part instructions.			
Points to own hair, shoes, nose and feet when requested.			

Social and Emotional Behaviour (Step 5)

Observation	Date first noted	Action Taken	Date Checked
Eats semi-solid food fed by adult.			
Able to feed self with fingers.			
Able to hold and drink from cup, using both hands.			
Able to hold spoon and feed independently.			
Takes off hat/socks/shoes.			
Gives notice of urgent need to go to the toilet.			
Accepts parents' absence by continuing activities.			
Plays alone contentedly.			

Play (Step 5)

Observation	Date first noted	Action Taken	Date Checked
As he stands, he enjoys pushing large wheeled toys and pulling toys on a string.			
Enjoys moving toys, blocks etc. from place to place in toy trucks.			
Becomes less easily bored. Throws toys around less and then usually as a result of annoyance or loss of interest.			
Copies other children at play as well as adults doing simple tasks.			
Enjoys playing with household objects, e.g. pans and brushes and playhouse replicas - simple pretend play.			
Is realising similarities and differences.			
Experiments with objects - squeezing and dropping them.			
Has begun to discover different properties of liquids and solids.			

Play (Step 5) - continued

Observation	Date first noted	Action Taken	Date Checked
Is competent at reaching out, grasping and letting go.			
Explores and experiments by moving around the room from object to object, looking, touching, tasting, smelling and listening.			
Hugs and carries doll or soft toy.			
Moves with music.			

Step 6
2 – 2½ years

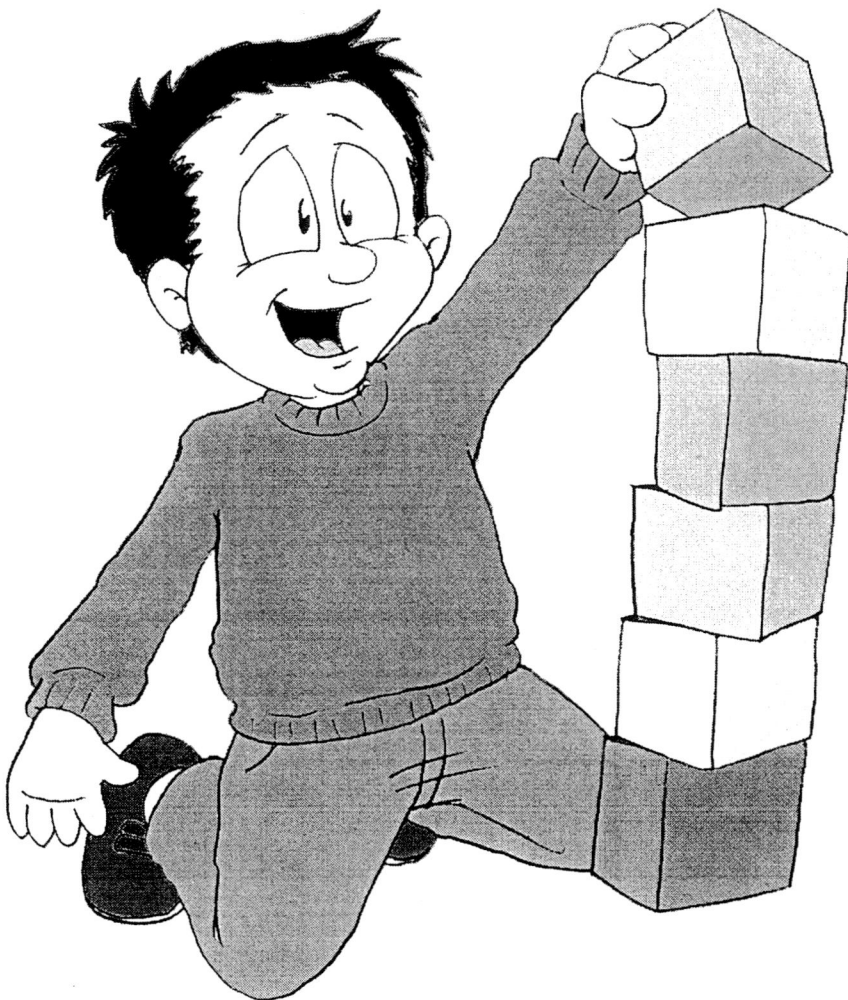

Posture and Large Movements (Step 6)

Observation	Date first noted	Action Taken	Date Checked
Runs safely, avoiding obstacles.			
Throws small ball overhand without falling.			
Kicks a large ball without falling.			
Squats to rest or play.			
Goes up - and needs help to come down - stairs, two feet to a step.			
Climbs a great deal.			
Moves wheeled toy by sitting on it and propelling backwards and forwards with feet.			

Vision and Fine Movements (Step 6)

Observation	Date first noted	Action Taken	Date Checked
Able to unscrew things.			
Can unwrap sweets.			
Able to build a tower of six to seven bricks.			
Scribbles spontaneously, using circular movements, as well as to and fro and dots.			
Able to imitate vertical line.			
Enjoys looking at books and being read to.			
Turns pages of books.			
Able to recognise familiar adults in pictures.			
Hand preference more obvious.			
Able to turn door knobs.			

Hearing and Speech (Step 6)

Observation	Date first noted	Action Taken	Date Checked
Able to use 50+ recognisable words and understands many more.			
Uses two or three word phrases.			
Beginning to listen with obvious interest to speech not directly addressed to him.			
Knows own full name.			
Constantly questions - 'What?' 'Where?'			
Constantly asking names of people, objects etc..			
Points to hair, hand, feet, nose, eyes, mouth, when requested.			
Beginning to use pronouns (I, you, me, mine).			
Good use of plurals.			
Beginning to learn nursery rhymes by heart.			

Hearing and Speech (Step 6) - continued

Observation	Date first noted	Action Taken	Date Checked
Listens to simple story with much talk about pictures.			
Gives and names familiar objects/pictures, when requested.			
Lots of repetition.			
Talks to self while playing.			
Able to sing simple songs with actions.			

Social and Emotional Behaviour (Step 6)

Observation	Date first noted	Action Taken	Date Checked
Becoming more independent (but still clings to mum when frightened or tired).			
Finds it difficult to share things.			
Comes to adult for affection.			
Co-operates in familiar activities with adults.			
Tends to develop jealousy.			
Defends own possessions with vigour.			
Resentful of attention shown to other children, particularly by familiar adult.			
Intensely curious regarding surroundings - little understanding of common dangers.			
Tantrums when frustrated, but attention can be distracted.			

Play (Step 6)

Observation	Date first noted	Action Taken	Date Checked
Plays happily near other children but not with them			
Gives first name			
Physical play with push/pull toys.			
Seeks adult involvement in simple sequence of pretend play.			
Talks continuously to himself during play.			
Very interested in messy play.			
Explores materials in creative activities.			
Concepts are real and visible.			
Experiments with being 'other people'.			

Step 7
2½ – 3 years

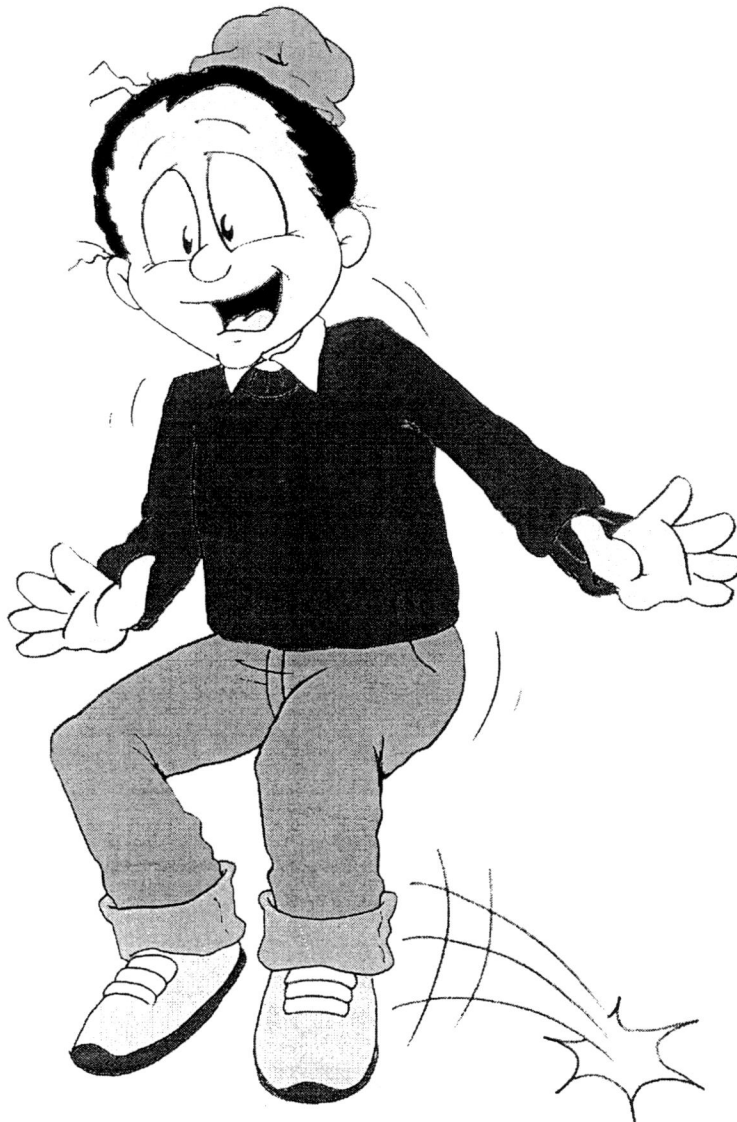

Posture and Large Movements (Step 7)

Observation	Date first noted	Action Taken	Date Checked
Walks upstairs confidently, two feet to a step.			
Walks downstairs holding rail, two feet to a step.			
Enjoys simple nursery apparatus.			
Can jump with two feet together.			
Able to stand on one foot and kick a ball.			
Stands on tip-toe.			
Pushes and pulls large toys with some skill.			

Vision and Fine Movements (Step 7)

Observation	Date first noted	Action Taken	Date Checked
Able to pick up tiny objects (e.g. needle, pins, threads) with one eye closed.			
Able to build a tower of seven or eight bricks.			
Recognises fine details when sharing picture books.			
Able to draw.			
Able to recognise picture of self.			
Able to thread large wooden beads with direction.			
Knows one colour.			
Holds pencil in preferred hand .			
Able to copy horizontal line and circle.			

Hearing and Speech (Step 7)

Observation	Date first noted	Action Taken	Date Checked
Still a certain amount or repetition.			
Able to use 200-300 words.			
Refers to self by name.			
Talks to himself a great deal.			
Responds to two-part instruction.			
Responds to questioning with talk.			
Enjoys simple familiar stories read from picture book.			
Able to recite a few simple nursery rhymes.			

Social and Emotional Behaviour (Step 7)

Observation	Date first noted	Action Taken	Date Checked
Fully toilet trained during the day.			
Pulls down pants at toilet but unable to replace.			
Can dress/undress himself to some degree.			
Eats well with spoon and possibly fork as well.			
Independent and rebellious.			
Less easily distracted.			
Emotionally still dependent on adults.			
Beginning to respond to less familiar adult, e.g. following simple instruction.			
Shares toys for short periods.			

Play (Step 7)

Observation	Date first noted	Action Taken	Date Checked
Imagination developing.			
Watches other children at play and occasionally joins in for a few minutes.			
Enjoys picture books and stories.			
Takes part in play which requires manipulative skills for short periods (inset puzzles, postboxes, etc.).			

Step 8
3 – 4 years

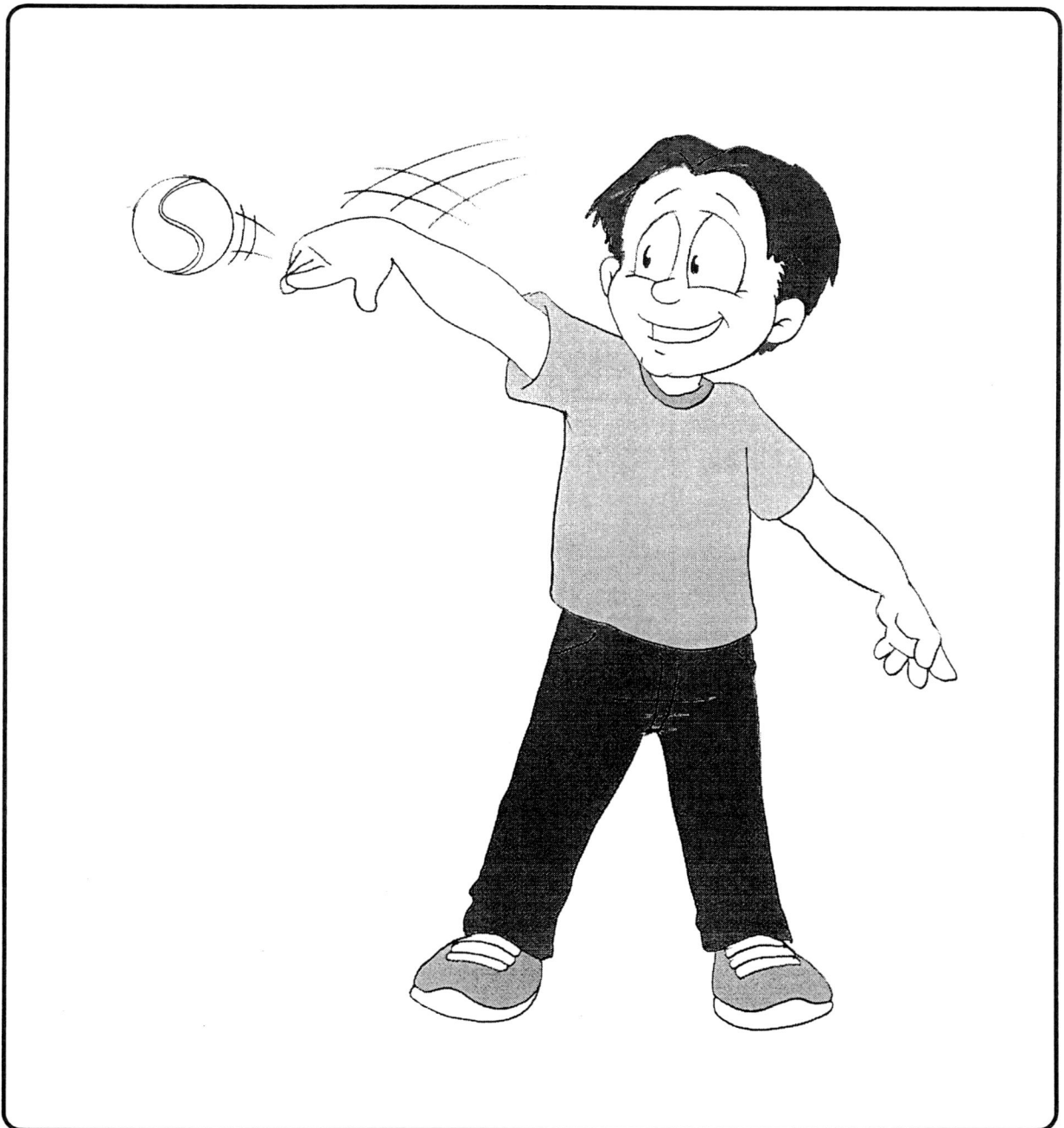

Posture and Large Movements (Step 8)

Observation	Date first noted	Action Taken	Date Checked
Stands on one foot momentarily.			
Goes upstairs with alternating feet.			
Jumps off bottom step with feet together.			
Able to pedal a tricycle.			
Able to avoid obstacles and turn corners while running.			
Can hop and walk a few steps on tip-toe.			
Catches large ball on or between extended arms.			
Kicks ball forcibly.			
Able to throw ball overhand competently.			

Vision and Fine Movements (Step 8)

Observation	Date first noted	Action Taken	Date Checked
Able to manipulate small objects with ease.			
Able to copy bridge of three bricks if shown.			
Able to build tower of nine bricks using two hands to steady.			
Able to thread large wooden beads on shoelace.			
Able to cut with scissors.			
Able to hold a pencil between first two fingers and thumb.			
Able to draw man consisting of head and one or two other features or parts.			
Matches primary colours.			
Enjoys painting with large brush on easel.			
Counts with adult to 3.			

Vision and Fine Movements (Step 8)

Observation	Date first noted	Action Taken	Date Checked
Helps adult count over 3.			
Joins in familiar number rhymes to 5.			

Hearing and Speech (Step 8)

Observation	Date first noted	Action Taken	Date Checked
Claps slowly in time to familiar rhymes.			
Enjoys moving to music and playing musical instruments.			
Large vocabulary (up to 1,000 words).			
Speech intelligible even to strangers.			
Speech modulating in loudness and range of pitch.			
Able to give full name and sex.			
Imagination very well developed.			
Chats to self in long monologues when playing.			
Very keen to tell news (sometimes stuttering in eagerness).			
Able to hold a conversation.			

Hearing and Speech (Step 8)

Observation	Date first noted	Action Taken	Date Checked
Can be reasoned with.			
Beginning to offer linguistic rather than physical resistance.			
Asks many questions (What? Where? Who?)			
Listens eagerly to favourite stories over and over again.			
Able to repeat (and sometimes sing) several nursery rhymes.			
Able to count by rote up to 10 but with little appreciation of quantity.			

Social and Emotional Behaviour (Step 8)

Observation	Date first noted	Action Taken	Date Checked
Able to use fork and spoon well.			
Beginning to develop table manners.			
Able to wash and dry own hands.			
Fully toilet trained (day and night).			
Able to pull pants down and up.			
Able to dress himself (except buttons and fastenings).			
General behaviour much improved - becoming more amenable.			
Likes to help with simple activities.			
More able to share toys and sweets.			
Able to think of others as well as himself.			

Social and Emotional Behaviour (Step 8) - continued

Observation	Date first noted	Action Taken	Date Checked
Co-operates in familiar activities with other children.			
Takes turns with play materials.			
Responds to reasoning with familiar adult.			
Makes a choice from a limited range of objects when asked.			
Shows some understanding of feelings by verbalising love, angry, sad, etc..			

Play (Step 8)

Observation	Date first noted	Action Taken	Date Checked
Shows evidence of imaginative play.			
Joins in active make-believe.			
Plays dressing up in adult clothes.			
Enjoys floor play with boxes, bricks etc.			
Seeks company of other children in physical play.			
Plays with construction toys, Lego, jigsaws for 10 minutes plus.			
Is beginning to understand abstract concepts.			
Is able to return to a game after a break.			
Fills and empties containers in sand/water play.			
Sorts and groups objects in small world play.			

Step 9
4 – 5 years

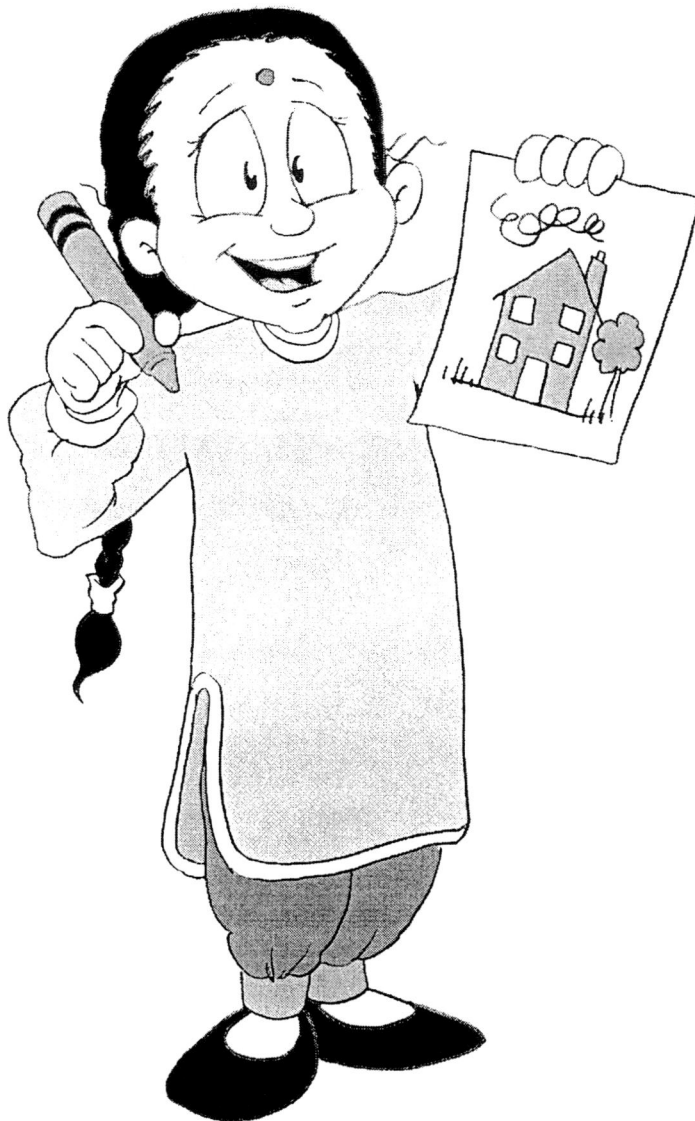

Posture and Large Movements (Step 9)

Observation	Date first noted	Action Taken	Date Checked
Balance nearly complete.			
Walks alone up and down stairs, one foot to a step.			
Able to climb ladders.			
Able to stand, walk and run on tip-toe.			
Able to sit with knees crossed.			
Shows increasing skill in ball games.			
Able to bend down to pick things up with straight legs.			
Able to balance on one foot for five seconds.			
Able to hop on preferred foot.			
Able to bring fingers in to touch nose, eyes closed.			

Vision and Fine Movements (Step 9)

Observation	Date first noted	Action Taken	Date Checked
Demonstrates even greater precision with small objects.			
Able to build a tower of 10 or more bricks.			
Able to build a bridge of three from model on request, or spontaneously.			
Able to hold and use pencil correctly, and with good control.			
Draws a man with head, trunk, legs and arms.			
Able to match red, yellow, blue and green (and sometimes name them).			
Able to draw simple house on request.			
Beginning to name drawings before production.			
Counts to five objects.			
Passes round cups (one each).			

Vision and Fine Movements (Step 9) - continued

Observation	Date first noted	Action Taken	Date Checked
Puts straws into bottles.			
Sorts colour, shape/animals.			

Hearing and Speech (Step 9)

Observation	Date first noted	Action Taken	Date Checked
Able to predict familiar events.			
Repetitions much reduced.			
Enjoys jokes and verbal incongruities.			
Able to count by rote to 20.			
Developing one to one correspondence up to four or five.			
Able to sing or repeat several nursery rhymes correctly.			
Listens to stories without pictures in large group of children.			
Able to name and describe familiar objects (size, colour, shape, function).			
Able to co-operate in games such as 'Simon Says'.			
Speech usually grammatically correct and intelligible.			

Hearing and Speech (Step 9) - continued

Observation	Date first noted	Action Taken	Date Checked
Articulation almost complete (sometimes r/w, y/l, d/th, k/t confusion).			
Able to recall the day's events.			
Able to give name, age and sex.			
Forever questioning (Why? When? How? and meanings of words).			
Enjoys listening to, and telling, long stories.			
Tends to confuse fact and fiction.			
Speech used more and more to control others.			
Becoming critical.			
Voice more subdued.			

Social and Emotional Behaviour (Step 9)

Observation	Date first noted	Action Taken	Date Checked
Able to wash himself competently.			
Enjoys playing with other children, although can be aggressive.			
General behaviour becoming more independent and self-willed.			
Confident enough to be impertinent at times.			
Understands reasons for doing and not doing things.			
Able to dress/undress (except ties and laces).			
Eats skillfully with spoon and fork.			
Showing sense of humour when talking or taking part in activities.			
Understands the need for taking turns.			

Social and Emotional Behaviour (Step 9) - continued

Observation	Date first noted	Action Taken	Date Checked
Understands the need to share.			
Shows sympathy for playmates in distress.			
Appreciates past, present and future.			
Has at least one identifiable friend.			
Usually uses 'please' and 'thank you'.			
Asks for help if in difficulty.			

Play (Step 9)

Observation	Date first noted	Action Taken	Date Checked
Sand and water play more sophisticated.			
Is able to put play skills to real use.			
Creates situations in small world play.			
Dramatic play evident in theme corner.			
Plays appropriately with toy telephone.			
Able to take part in simple rule-learning games (e.g. lotto, picture dominoes).			
Takes part in complex imaginative play with improvised props.			
Constructive outside building with any materials available.			

Step 10
5 years

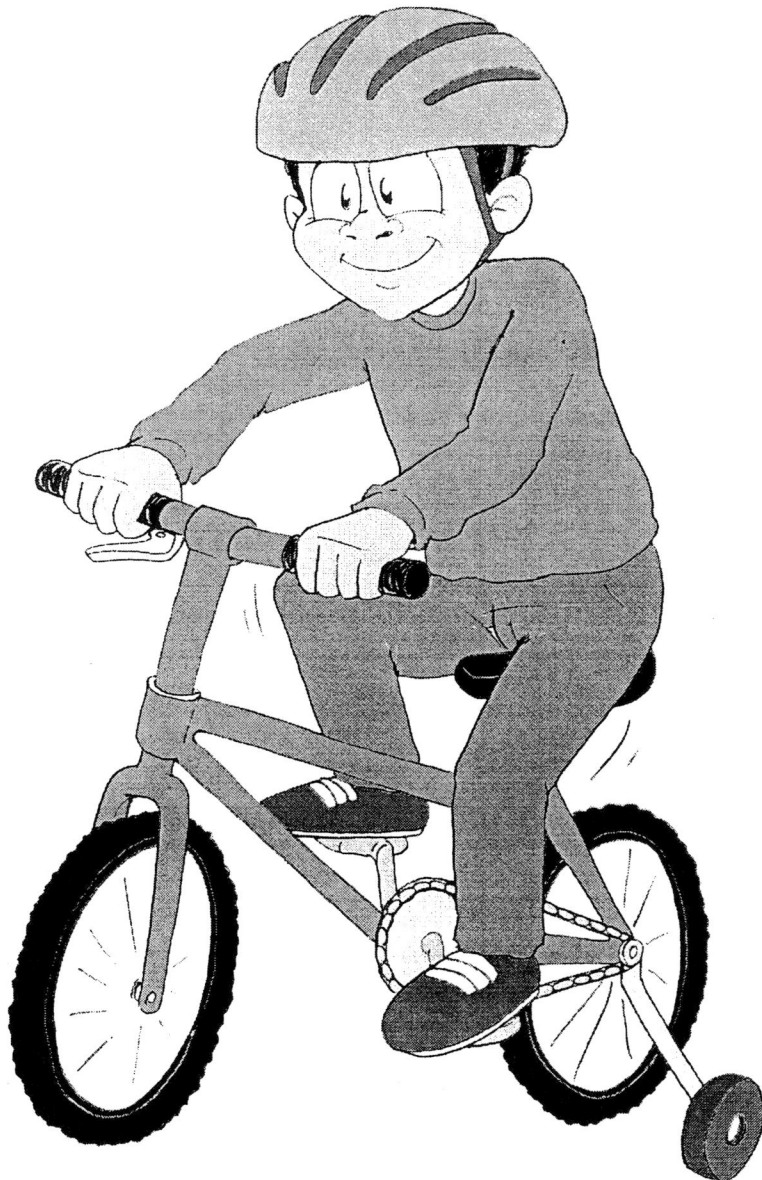

Posture and Large Movements (Step 10)

Observation	Date first noted	Action Taken	Date Checked
Able to walk on narrow line.			
Able to run on tip-toe.			
Able to balance on one foot with arms folded for 5+ seconds.			
Able to skip on alternate feet.			
Able to hop on both left and right feet.			
Moves rhythmically to music.			
Strong grip with either hand.			
Plays all ball games with considerable ability.			
Can ride a bicycle.			

Posture and Large Movements (Step 10) - continued

Observation	Date first noted	Action Taken	Date Checked
Active and skillful in climbing, sliding, swinging etc..			
Able to jump over an object 25 cm high.			

Vision and Fine Movements (Step 10)

Observation	Date first noted	Action Taken	Date Checked
Able to draw house with door, windows , roof and chimney.			
Able to draw many pictures spontaneously, each containing several items.			
Able to count fingers of one hand with index finger of other.			
Able to copy numbers 1-10.			
Able to count objects to 10 (sometimes to 20)			
Able to name red, yellow, green and blue.			
Able to match 10 colours or more.			
Able to tie shoelaces.			
Able to tell which pile of counters has 'more' and prove it.			
Able to thread large needle alone.			

Vision and Fine Movements (Step 10) - continued

Observation	Date first noted	Action Taken	Date Checked
Able to sew real stitches.			
Has good control in writing and drawing (pencils/paint brushes).			
Able to copy ○ □ △			
Able to write a few letters spontaneously.			
Able to copy/write own first name.			
Able to copy/write simple words.			
Able to draw recognisable man with head, trunk, legs, arms, fingers, feet and features.			
Able to colour neatly, staying within outline.			

Hearing and Speech (Step 10)

Observation	Date first noted	Action Taken	Date Checked
Speech fluent and grammatically correct.			
Uses compound sentences. (I spilt my drink and it went on my picture.)			
Able to define concrete nouns by use, e.g. pencil to draw, car to drive.			
Enjoys being read to or told stories.			
Acts out stories in detail.			
Able to invent a short story.			
Able to recite poems and sing nursery rhymes.			
Enjoys jokes and riddles.			
Has ear for detail.			
Able to appreciate rhythm and rhyme.			

Hearing and Speech (Step 10) - continued

Observation	Date first noted	Action Taken	Date Checked
Able to give name, age, address, sex and birthday.			
Able to give opposites to familiar words.			
Asks meaning of abstract words and attempts to use them.			
Knows what day of the week it is.			
Answers questions with a sentence.			
Uses language to reason. (Why? ... because ... If ... then ...)			

Social and Emotional Behaviour (Step 10)

Observation	Date first noted	Action Taken	Date Checked
Picks up an object dropped nearby, without being asked.			
Understands the need for order and tidiness (may need constant reminders).			
Usually asks permission to use someone else's possessions/equipment.			
Will go to the aid of another child in distress.			
Shows tenderness towards younger children and pets.			
Senses disapproval and reacts by changing behaviour.			
Is now capable of being independent.			
Knows about rules of fair play (has learned to cheat).			
Is quite competitive.			
Can manage knife and fork.			

Social and Emotional Behaviour (Step 10) - continued

Observation	Date first noted	Action Taken	Date Checked
Has become more sensible and controlled.			
Chooses own friends.			
Shows definite sense of humour.			
Understands meaning of clock-time in relation to daily programme.			

Play (Step 10)

Observation	Date first noted	Action Taken	Date Checked
Domestic and dramatic play continued from day to day.			
Floor games very complicated.			
Plans and builds constructively indoors and outdoors.			
Able to complete interlocking jigsaws.			
Able to complete play-tray jigsaw.			
Shows enthusiasm and some degree of understanding in design and technology projects.			

Observation	Date first noted	Action Taken	Date Checked

Suggested resources

Posture and large movements

Some suggested activities for developing skills:

Baby bouncer

Bouncing cradle

Crawling activities, progressing to:
- *unilateral* (moving arm and leg on one side of body together)
- *cross lateral* (right arm with left leg and *vice versa*)

Push-along toys

Climbing in and out of cardboard boxes

Simple obstacle courses

Outside play – climbing frames, slide, swing, trampoline, see-saw, benches, hoops, pedal cars, bikes and tricycles, etc.

Skipping games

Play tunnels/cubes

Hopscotch

Stepping stones

Traffic lights

Follow-my-leader

Trips to the park

Ball games – football, catch, etc.

Vision and fine movements

Some suggested activities for developing skills

Mobiles

Activity centres

Play mats

Activity gyms

Waterballs

Stacking toys

Shape-sorting toys

Pop-up games

Sharing books with adult

Play-dough

Finger painting/foot painting

Threading activities – cotton reels, buttons, beads, pasta, etc.

Peg-boards/unifix pattern trays

Cutting activities

Finger rhymes

Colouring – starting with large, simple shape

Odd-one-out

Find the same/Snap

Construction apparatus – Duplo/Stickle bricks

Kim's Game

Gluing and sticking activities

Painting/printing activities – using a variety of materials

Sequencing/pattern repetition

Matching/sorting activities – shape, colour, size, texture

Pre-writing activities (see *Towards Handwriting*, available from The Questions Publishing Company.)

Hearing and speech

Some suggested activities for developing skills

Rattles

Musical instruments – shakers, drums, triangles, etc.

Feely bag/box

Nursery rhymes/action rhymes

Sharing books – and discussion of content

Blowing bubbles, balloons, racing ping-pong balls

Good role model and positive guidance for correct speech/grammar

Message taking

Using senses (taste, smell, touch, hearing, sight)

Using different texture, materials, etc. (pasta/sticks/tissue paper/ cotton wool/leaves/feathers)

Encouragement to expand answers to more than a single word

'I went to the shops and I bought . . .'

Chinese Whispers

Sequencing pictures and telling story

Riddles

Retelling of favourite stories

Use of puppets/masks to dramatise stories

Encouraging adult visitors to stimulate conversation (policeman/ lollipop lady/theatre groups/animal man etc.)

Picture/sound matching games

Stories using taped sounds

Re-telling the past ('What did we do last time?')

Going for a walk/looking at surroundings

Social and emotional behaviour

Some suggested activities for developing skills

Teddies/soft toys

Books/jigsaws/picture cards showing a variety of emotions/feelings

Social interaction – sitting at table, taking turns, etc.

Collaborative play

Simple role play

Simple rules to be followed by *everyone* in the nursery

Encouragement to seek help and guidance (from adults and peers)

Provision of good role model and positive guidance

Following simple instructions

Encouragement for independence (toilet, clothes, eating, etc.)

Support in development of sense of self-worth

Making choices (in play/discussion and in real life)

Play

Some suggested activities for developing skills

Peek-a-boo

Pat-a-cake

Playmats

Finger puppets

Dressing-up clothes

Home corner – dolls, teddies, furniture, prams, cots, etc.

Shopping trolley and play foods

Pretend shop

Puppet theatre

Large cardboard boxes – just waiting to be turned into boats, tables, shops, etc.

Masks

Role-play activities

Telephones

Paddling pool and toys

Face painting

Sand and water play

Large construction toys – bricks etc.

Model zoo/farm animals

Train set

Model cars

Jigsaws

Playground games, e.g. *Farmer's In His Den, Hokey Cokey, Hopscotch*

Simple collaborative games – throwing, rolling, catching games

References

From Birth To Five Years
Mary Sheridan (1993) Routledge, London.

Before Alpha
Beve Hornsby (1995) Souvenir Press Ltd.

Early Learning Assessment And Development
Audrey Curtis and Mary Wignall (1982) Thomas Nelson.

Portage Checklist
Staffordshire Portage

Checklist For Reception Age Children
S.N.I.P.

Playladders
Hannah Mortimer

Denver Development Screening Test
Premier Health

Towards Handwriting
The Questions Publishing Company Ltd/Staffordshire
SENSS Enterprises